The Detox Diet
Plan Guide for Beginners

How to Lose Weight Fast to
Optimize Your Health, Revitalize
Your Appearance & Rapidly
Increase Your Energy Through
Detox Cleanses

Joel Jackson

Wait! Before You Read Any Further...Are You On A Diet or Really Want to Lose A Few Extra Pounds?

If your answer was YES, then you are not alone. A majority of people are wanting to lose 5, 10, 20 or even 50 pounds! However, a lot of us don't know how and resort to extreme dieting or starvation.

Fortunately, you have found the right place! Check out your FREE bonus to keep you motivated to complete your goal and then learn how you can rid your body of the unwanted weight!

Free Bonus

As a gift to you, I'd like to offer you a FREE BONUS to enjoy. Use the motivation from this video to propel you forward to reach your goals!

Detox Diet FREE BONUS GUIDE!

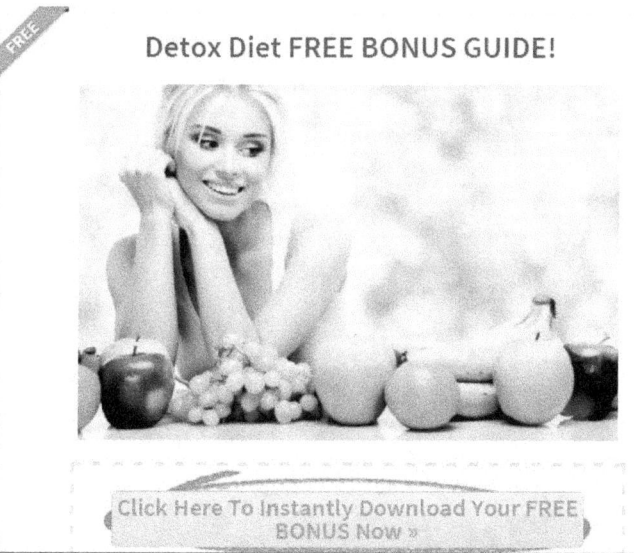

Click Here To Instantly Download Your FREE BONUS Now »

In addition to subscribing, you will receive notification when my other books are available for free and helpful resources and tools that you can use in your health journey!

Thank you so much for subscribing. I look forward to sharing more resources with you.

Here's the link you need to manually copy into your address bar

https://joypublishing.leadpages.net/detox-cleanse/

Table Of Contents

Introduction

I want to thank you and congratulate you for purchasing the book, "Detox Diet Plan Guide for Beginners: How to Lose Weight Fast to Optimize Your Health, Revitalize Your Appearance & Rapidly Increase Your Energy Through Detox Cleanses."

This book contains proven steps and strategies on how to have an over-all sense of well-being and increase your energy levels by doing the detox diet.

This book also features some examples of detox diet programs which were actually used and made popular by celebrities such as Beyonce Knowles, Gwyneth Paltrow and singer Ashanti.

Thanks again for purchasing this book, I hope you enjoy it! Please take some time to stop by and LIKE our Facebook page:

https://www.facebook.com/joypublishing

With gratitude,

Joel Jackson

Chapter 1: Detox Diet – The Basics

Detox is short for "detoxification", which refers to the process of eliminating the toxic substances outside the body. A detox diet simply implies that you are getting rid of harmful toxins from your intestines, kidneys, liver and the bloodstream through a strict diet.

One of the objectives of a detox diet is to eliminate the harmful toxins inside the body. These harmful substances that we ingest and breathe everyday can cause diseases, fatigue, headaches and skin problems. The main objective of a detox diet is to help the body get back to its clean, healthy state. Toxin elimination is believed to purify the body organs and help them to function more efficiently.

Detox diet plans have been around for many centuries. Detox diets have been widely known for its beneficial effects. A detox diet plan is a low-calorie, mostly liquid, diet strategy which helps cleanse the body. While there are a lot of various detox diets with different specific objectives, including Martha's Vineyard Detox Diet and the Fruit Flush, the general idea behind all of them is just the same.

What is a Detox Diet Plan?

The detox diet plan is deemed to be very restrictive. The detox diet requires the dieter to give up a lot of food items that contain certain ingredients believed to be toxins. Since the detox diet plan is very restrictive, experts suggest dieters to use it for only a short period of time. It is also wise to make sure that you are not experiencing any pressing health issues that may be aggravated by such a restrictive diet.

While there are a lot of detox diet plans out there, the most basic detox diet involves three (3) days of water fasting and another 10 days of a monotrophic diet. The monotrophic diet is where you put a limit to yourself to a single type of fruit every meal. However, in between lunch and dinner, some detox diet plans can allow a huge glass of carrot juice.

The detox diet plan should be strictly adhered to for 13 days. After which, you should ease into a normal eating plan by consuming strictly raw food.

In addition to the food regimen, there are some types of detox diets that will suggest the dieter to take time every day to undergo a complete body cleansing. There are a number of ways to boost the beneficial effects of your detox diet plan. It can be through the use of saunas, baths or herbs. There are even some types detox diet plans which recommend the use of enemas or laxatives to aid in the process.

The Benefits of a Detox Diet

1. Enhanced sense of overall wellbeing

    Detoxifying will make you feel good about yourself. Detoxifying is usually used strategically to reduce weight or jump-start a new diet plan. However, there really is no greater reason than just to feel good. When you set the stage for overall wellbeing, you are going to improve every aspect of your life. You should expect to see a renewed zest for life, better productivity at work and better relationships.

2. Feeling lighter

The process of detoxification or cleansing will make a person feel lighter. There are a number of reasons why this is the case, particularly if the dieter is doing a colon cleanse as part of the regimen. When you avoid eating foods that cause you to feel bloated and substitute them with fresh organic foods and vegetables, you will notice that you feel lighter.

3. Shinier and clearer skin

A detox diet does not only make one feel better. It actually can help in making a person look better. Eliminating all the toxins in the body can make clear up your skin. It can also make the hair look shinier. When people see you after a detox, do not be surprised if they will be complimenting how good you look.

4. Enhanced mental focus

Undertaking a detox program can boost your mental focus. If you eliminate all harmful toxins from your body, you'll have better focus and be more creative and productive at work.

5. Strengthened immune system

A boost in your immune system is one of the most amazing benefits of undergoing a detox. After eliminating your body's harmful toxins, you will notice that you've become healthier and less prone to illnesses. Your body will be well equipped to combat all types of illnesses and diseases.

6. Increased levels of energy

   Having a lot of toxic materials in the body can affect your energy levels. You may start to feel lethargic and sluggish. Instead of participating in various activities or going out with your friends, you will probably just want to lie down on the couch the whole day. If you undertake a detox, your energy levels will boost. Eventually, you'll feel new and energized to do more activities.

7. Eliminate excessive wastes

   Excess toxic materials can weigh you down and make you feel lethargic. When you undertake a detox regimen, your colon will be cleansed and excess toxins will be rid from your body.

Chapter 2: What are Some Examples of Detox Foods?

What To Eat During Detox

Apples

Apples are rich in essential nutrients. This fruit is abundant in minerals, vitamins, fiber as well as beneficial phytochemicals such terpenoids, flavonoids, D-Glucarate. These compounds are utilized in the process of detoxifying. Phlorizidin, a type of flavonoid, is believed to help in the stimulation of bile production, which aids in the detox process as the liver eliminates toxic materials through the bile. Apples are also abundant of pectin, a type of soluble fiber. Pectin can help in getting rid of heavy metals and additives found inside the body. It is suggested to eat only fresh organic apples as the non-organic varieties are found to be abundant in pesticide residues.

Turmeric

The spice turmeric is found to contain curcumin, its active ingredient and is responsible for its yellow color. The rate which the detox pathways work will depend on the person's lifestyle, age, genes and the amount of good nutrients involved in the detox process. Curcumin is widely utilized in Ayurvedic medicine as a cure for liver and digestive disorders.

Artichoke

Aside from being tasty, artichokes are also amazingly healthy. They have been reported to boost the production of bile and protect and purify the liver. Artichokes also have a gentle diuretic effect on the kidneys, which ensures the proper elimination of toxic wastes once the liver has broken them down.

Garlic

Garlic should always be present in every detox diet plan. Garlic has powerful antibiotic, antiseptic and antiviral properties. Eliminating pathogenic microorganisms can reduce the amount of toxic wastes produced inside the body. Garlic contains essential sulphuric substances which makes it a powerful detoxifier.

Lemons

Lemon is a potent fruit that releases enzymes and converts toxins into a water-soluble form, which can be readily eliminated out of the body. Drinking lemon water every morning will aid in neutralizing the pH balance in the digestive system. To enhance toxin elimination, you may also add ground flaxseeds.

Flaxseed

Flaxseeds serve a lot of different purposes. When undergoing a detox process, it is important that the toxic materials in the body are excreted properly. Ground flaxseed is abundant in fiber, which helps bind and eliminate toxic wastes from the intestinal tract. Flaxseeds are also a potent source of essential omega 3 fatty acids. Try taking 2 tablespoons of ground flaxseed combined with lemon water daily.

Broccoli Sprouts

Broccoli is among the powerful vegetables in the brassica family. It contains essential phytochemicals that are released whenever digested, cooked, fermented, chewed or chopped. The potent substances are released and broken down into D-glucarate, indole-3-carbinol and sulphorophanes, which all participates in the detox process. Broccoli sprouts can actually result to more benefits than regular broccoli. They have 20 times more sulfurophane. Broccoli sprouts may be added to salads.

Sea Vegetables

Usually referred to as seaweeds, sea vegetables are potent antioxidants that assist in alkalizing the blood and strengthening the digestive tract. Seaweeds contain algin, which absorbs toxic materials from the digestive tract like how a water softener softens tap water.

Beetroot

Beets are abundant sources of beta-carotene, vitamins b3, b6 and C. Beets are also potent sources of calcium, zinc, magnesium and iron – all of which are necessary to promote effective elimination and detoxification of waste materials. Beets also promote good liver and gallbladder health. These are organs that play significant roles in breaking down and eliminating toxins. The high amount of fiber found in this potent food enhances digestion and aids in eliminating body waste.

What to Avoid During Detox

When on a detox diet plan, make sure to avoid following foods:

- Squashes and fizzy drinks, including diet versions

- Salt

- Mayonnaise, store-bought salad dressing, pickles and sauces

- Coffee and tea

- Alcohol

- Takeaways, ready-made sauces, ready meals and processed foods

- Sugar, jam, sweets and chocolate

- Savoury and crisp snacks including salted nuts

- Any type of food that contains wheat such as battered foods, quiche, pastry, pies, biscuits, cakes, cereals, croissants and bread

- Margarine and butter

- Cream, eggs, cheese and milk

- Meat products such as pate, burgers and sausages

- Turkey, chicken and red meat

Chapter 3: Sample 3-day Detox Diet Plan

This healthy 3-day detox diet plan does not involve deprivation or fasting. Instead of following an extreme detox diet plan that restricts just about every type of food except vegetables and fruit, this plan is safer and a better alternative. This healthy detox diet plan will leave you with the essential nutrients your body needs if you follow it for three (3) days:

Day 1

Breakfast:

Fruit salad with yoghurt, sprinkled with oats

Lunch:

Mediterranean salad with rice cakes

Directions:

Serve rice cakes with black pepper, fresh basil, tomatoes, avocado and rocket. A handful of unsalted nuts may also be used

Snack:

Plain popcorn

Dinner:

Potato Bean casserole

Direction: Lightly fry a selection of commonly used casserole vegetables such as parsnip, carrots and onion in a little olive oil with garlic. Add diced potato and fry for a short while. Mix in your favorite beans, black pepper and fresh vegetable stock.

Day 2

Breakfast:

Muesli and yoghurt
Directions: Make homemade muesli with dried fruit, nuts, seeds and oats. Serve with yoghurt.

Lunch:

Tuna with sweet corn jacket potato served with salad

Directions: Top jacket potato with tuna. Mix with natural yogurt and sweet corn. Serve with salad.

Snack:

Natural yogurt combined with honey

Dinner:

Sweet and sour stir fry with rice

Directions: Lightly fry a selection of chopped vegetables including mushrooms, baby sweet corn, peppers and onions. Mix in honey, white wine vinegar, tomato puree, canned tomatoes and canned pineapple.

Day 3

Breakfast:

Yogurt with fresh fruit, sweetened with honey

Lunch:

Vegetable soup and oatcakes

Directions:

Prepare a big bowl of homemade or supermarket "fresh" lentil or vegetable soup with oatcakes

Snack:

Handful of unsalted seeds or nuts

Dinner:

Baked salmon with jacket potato

Directions: Bake salmon fillet and serve with steamed vegetables along with jacket potato

Chapter 4: Popular Detox Diets That You Should Try

The body is exposed to a lot of toxic substances every day – from alcohol to air pollution. These harmful substances accumulate in the body; such buildup leads to different types of sickness, fatigue and bloating. Supposedly, detox diets get rid of these harmful substances and thus making the body healthier.

So why are detox diets very popular these days? It is not only because of the claimed health benefit, but because of the weight reduction effects. Following are some examples of detox diets popularized by celebrities such as Beyonce Knowles and Gwyneth Paltrow.:

1. The Master Cleanse

    The Master cleanse was invented in 1941 by Stanley Burroughs. The Master Cleanse is a liquid diet which became a household name in 2006 when Beyonce Knowles reported to lose 20 pounds for her role in the movie "Dreamgirls". The Master Cleanse is also known as the Lemon Diet or the Maple Syrup Diet. It involves consuming up to 12 glasses of a special beverage prepared every day for about 10 to 45 days. The Master Cleanse is probably the most popular detox diet plan out there.

    The Master Cleanse concoction is made with cayenne pepper, maple syrup and lemon juice. Reportedly, each of the ingredients serves a particular purpose as follows:

    Cayenne pepper – added boost in metabolism

Maple syrup – for an added energy boost and flavor

Lemon juice – cleanses the body

In addition to consuming the master cleanse concoction, the process also involves the use of laxative every day. The master cleanse is a very restrictive diet that will surely result to weight reduction.

Who's used the master cleanse detox diet? In addition to Beyonce Knowles, who once referred to the diet saying: "I was very hungry, therefore I was evil". There were other celebrities who have forced down this lemony concoction. Celebrities who've used the master cleanse detox diet include Demi Moore and Ashton Kutcher, singer Ashanti, Howard Stern's assistant Robin Quivers and magician David Blaine.

2. The Cabbage Soup Diet

This detox diet plan involves consuming a bottomless bowl of cabbage soup. On the diet regimen, dieters are allowed to consume all the cabbage soup they want for seven days. They may also eat a few other select foods including skim milk, vegetable and fruits.

Cabbage is very abundant in dietary fiber, which aids in cleansing the digestive system and reportedly detoxifies the body. The cabbage soup diet claims a 10-pound weight reduction in only a week's time. The Cabbage soup diet is also a very restrictive one; thereby weight loss is the inevitable result.

So who has used the cabbage soup diet? Jaime Pressley has committed herself to eat unlimited cabbage soup to get rid of unwanted baby weight. Bill Clinton has reportedly used the cabbage soup diet to slim down in preparation for his daughter's wedding.

3. Clean Program

The Clean Program was invented by Alejandro Junger. This detox diet regimen claims to cleanse and depuff the body by avoiding gluten as well as some of the most common types of allergen from one's diet. While undergoing the diet regimen, dieters are allowed to eat one solid meal daily, drink two liquid meals and take supplements.

Dr. Junger suggests that detoxers solid meals for lunch since the overnight fast will aid to free up energy for the detoxification process. In addition to this, Dr. Junger says that the solid meal must be sugar-free, processed foods and dairy products. In addition to the restricted diet, dieters are also required to take herbal laxatives. The supplements and shakes are already provided by the program. The 21- Day Ultimate Clean Program kit is sold for $350.

So who has used the clean program? Dona Karan swears by the clean program. Gwyneth Paltrow uses the clean program at least twice a year, while Demi Moore recently tried this program after quitting the Master Cleanse detox diet.

4. Martha's Vineyard Detox Diet

The Martha's Vineyard Detox Diet is also popularly known as the "Lose 21 Pounds in 21 Days Diet". This diet regimen requires the dieter to consume specialized vegetable and fruit liquids. Also consumed are some solid vegetables which are supposedly the mixture of these vegetables, supplements and fruit drinks which cleanses up the body. This diet regimen was invented by Roni deLuz, who is a nurse. She said she designed this restrictive liquid diet when she was trying to heal herself.

This program allows the dieter to choose between a 2-day, 7-day or 21-day plan which all involves taking a special liquid every 2 hours. DeLuz suggests a 21-day detox to be done annually, a 7-day clean up for every season and a 2-day detox every weekend. In principle, once the body is rid of toxic materials, it will be able to function well, allowing the metabolism to soar and promote weight reduction.

So who has actually used this diet regimen? Angelina Jolie is said to have undertaken this detox diet regimen to reduce weight for a certain movie role.

5. The Ultimate Tea diet

This popular detox diet was invented by Mark Ukra, who is one of the world's leading tea experts. According to Ukra, tea promotes detoxification and weight reduction, mainly because of its three potent ingredients: Caffeine, which stimulates thermogenesis, a bodily process used to generate energy from digesting food; it has appetite suppression and diuretic properties which helps in getting rid of toxins through the kidney; L-theanine, which also has appetite suppression properties and counters caffeine's harmful effects; and **EGCG, which enhances the body's fat burning efficiency.**

Chapter 5: Detox Diet Frequently Asked Questions (FAQs)

Following are some of the most frequently asked questions (FAQs) about detox diet:

1. What is a detox?

    Detox or detoxify is also commonly referred to as cleansing. Basically, detox is a process by which an individual undertakes a program, commonly involving some diet modification or supplement to the diet, to help in getting rid toxic materials and parasites from the body that can accumulate in the body over time.

    Unfortunately, we live in a society where there are a lot of potentially dangerous substances everywhere. These harmful substances can be in our homes, restaurants, shops, and offices. Our bodies are constantly getting rid of these harmful substances through sweat, bowel movements, urine and breathing.

    However, many toxic materials still remain inside the body, either stuck in the organs and intestines or fat cells. It is very important to help the body from time to time to get rid of these harmful substances. A detox/cleansing diet should be done at least once a year to help the body get rid of the harmful toxic substances.

2. Will I feel better after undergoing a detox or cleanse diet regimen?

You will definitely feel the difference between before and after undergoing a detox diet regimen. If necessary, you should also improve your exercise for more optimal results.

3. Will I experience any side effects while undergoing a detox diet regimen?

When you are trying to eliminate the toxic materials from the body too many get eliminated into the blood stream. A dieter may get an occasional stomachache or headache, or even feel emotional. Keep in mind that all of these are part of the process.

You may have taken a long period of time to accumulate all the toxic materials in your body. Do not expect you will be able to eliminate all of them at once. It may take a few weeks or months in order to achieve optimal results.

4. What kind of parasites or toxins that I likely have in my body?

Almost everyone who lives in a populated area will have toxic materials in their bodies. This is just normal.

Clinical studies have reported that the human body is a great host to several other organisms such as bacteria. Some of these bacterial organisms are harmless and, in fact, aid in the process of digestion. However, there are also some types of bad bacteria that can enter into the body. Aside from bacteria, there are also intestinal flukes, liver flukes and worms of different types that can enter the body.

5. Can I entirely get rid of these parasites by undergoing a detox diet?

While undergoing a detox regimen will help in getting rid of toxic materials and parasites inside the body, unfortunately, they will always be present. The good news is that, you can actually do quite a lot in order to lessen the chances of getting them back into your body.

Try to stop putting your fingers near your mouth or biting your nails, particularly when you have made contact with meat, soil, pets or other areas that may contain parasites.

Free Bonus

As a gift to you, I'd like to offer you a FREE BONUS to enjoy. Use the motivation from this video to propel you forward to reach your goals!

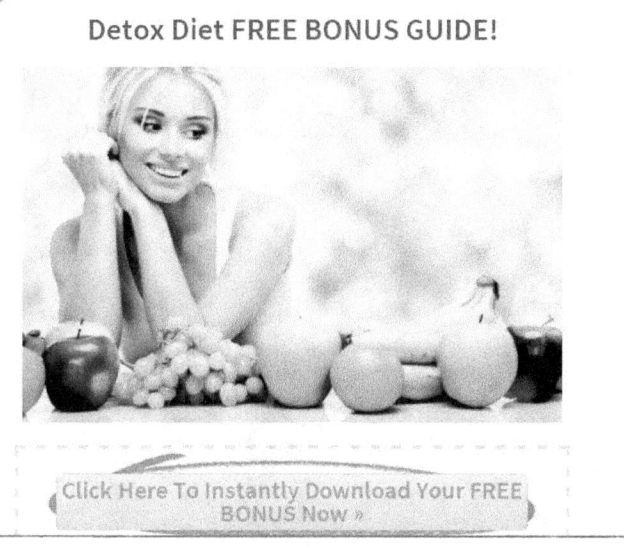

Detox Diet FREE BONUS GUIDE!

Click Here To Instantly Download Your FREE BONUS Now »

In addition to subscribing, you will receive notification when my other books are available for free and helpful resources and tools that you can use in your health journey!

Thank you so much for subscribing. I look forward to sharing more resources with you.

Here's the link you need to manually copy into your address bar

https://joypublishing.leadpages.net/detox-cleanse/

Conclusion

Thank you again for purchasing this book!

I hope this book was able to help you to have a deeper understanding of what a detox diet is and its many health benefits.

The next step is to try a specific detox diet regimen that you are most interested with or try the sample 3-day detox diet plan as featured in this book.

Finally, if you enjoyed this book, please take the time to share your thoughts and post a positive review. It'd be greatly appreciated!

Also, remember to download your FREE BONUS VIDEO!

In addition, please remember to LIKE our Facebook page in order to find other resources and upcoming promotions:

https://www.facebook.com/joypublishing

With sincere thanks,

Joel Jackson

One Last Thing...

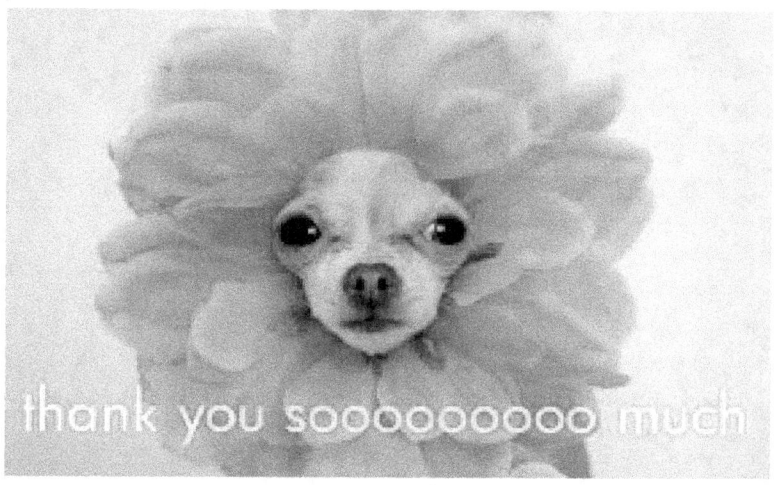

thank you sooooooooo much

If you believe that this book is worth sharing, would you please take the time to let others know how it affected your life? If it turns out to make a difference in the lives of others, they will be forever grateful to you, as will I.